CARB CYCLING

By Julia Bond

The trademarks that are used are without any consent, and the publication of the trademark is without permission or backing by the trademark owner. All trademarks and brands within this book are for clarifying purposes only and are the owned by the owners themselves, not affiliated with this document.

Disclaimer and Terms of Use: The Author and Publisher has strived to be as accurate and complete as possible in the creation of this book, notwithstanding the fact that he does not warrant or represent at any time that the contents within are accurate due to the rapidly changing nature of the Internet. While all attempts have been made to verify information provided in this publication, the Author and Publisher assumes no responsibility for errors, omissions, or contrary interpretation of the subject matter herein.

Any perceived slights of specific persons, peoples, or organizations are unintentional. In practical advice books, like anything else in life, there are no guarantees of results. Readers are cautioned to rely on their own judgment about their individual circumstances and act accordingly.

This book is not intended for use as a source of legal, medical, business, accounting or financial advice. All readers are advised to seek services of competent professionals in the legal, medical, business, accounting, and finance fields.

TABLE OF CONTENTS

INTRODUCTION

Carb Cycling is exactly as it sounds- cycling your carbs. You may remember the "low-carb" diet that was a national fad several years ago. People saw results, for a while at least. The main problem with low-carb diets is that they are meant as temporary diets- you cannot eat that way forever. Your body can't eat that way, as it needs carbs for daily function. Yes, believe it or not, your body requires carbs.

Then there's the opposite end of the spectrum, those who advocate high- carb diets. While high-carb diets help to speed your metabolism, they are not ideal for weight-loss, as there is not a sufficient deficit to help you shed the pounds. This is where carb-cycling comes in.

While many fad diets claim to "reset" your body, all they do is drain the water, nutrients, and vitamins from your body for quick weight loss, without being able to continue it. Carb cycling literally resets your body by breaking all of those bad habits you have developed, while at the same time teaching your body new, better habits. It's a simple, one-step process and a great plan for a lifetime of health. Carb cycling is easy, inexpensive and you can do it all on your own- there is no need to spend lots of money on a program or special foods. There are resources you can purchase to help you on your journey, but you can succeed without these as well.

The "magic" of carb cycling is that is works by giving your body both the fuel it needs to increase metabolism, and creating calorie deficits to increase fat loss. Days are rotated between high-carb days, and low-carb days. Did you know your body is designed to eat more than three meals a day? Three meals was not a common occurrence until the industrial age. Rather, to maximize weight loss and keep your metabolism burning, the best schedule is one that eats five times a day, or every three hours. This may sound like a lot, but after a few days of eating this way, your body will become hungry and want to eat every three hours. Eating three meals a day will be a struggle, as it is a lot of food especially early in the day but, it wil work. This combined with pre-portioned meals and a regular exercise routine, including cardio and weight training, will burn fat and tone muscle!

CARB CYCLING - THE SECRET TO HEALTHY WEIGHT LOSS

It is not uncommon to hear people complain that diets do not work for them. Most diets force you to eat only fruits and vegetables or to replace meals with energy drinks. The reason many of these diets do not work is because they focus on making money and not actually helping you to lose weight. What many people do not know is there is a science behind losing weight effectively and keeping it off. Many diets ignore this fact and so, they do not work. Carb cycling is a way of eating that focuses on the science behind losing weight.

Catabolism is process the body goes through that produces fat in the body and anabolism helps the body to build muscle. Many diets only focus on catabolism; so many people are never given the chance to rebuild muscle. By carb cycling, you alternate the days in which you eat the normal amount of carbohydrates and the days when very little carbs are taken in. The process works because on the low carb days, a calorie deficit is created and the regular carb days keep the metabolism from slowing down and the body from gaining weight.

On regular carb days, it is recommended you eat 350-400 grams of carbohydrates. This is not too difficult because it is about the normal amount. However, it is important to distinguish between good carbs and bad ones. You will want to try to stick to unrefined carbs that can be found in whole grains and fruits. The added bonus to these carbohydrates is that they can also help fight off bacteria and diseases. The second part of carb cycling is the low carb days. On these days, try to keep your carb count under 300 grams and stay away from foods with flour or sugar.

With the carb rotation diet, it is not necessary to starve or ever feel hungry. It is important to keep track of the days of the cycle however, because it can be easy to make a mistake and confuse the low carb and regular carb days. Make sure you are eating the right type of carbohydrates and during the optimal eating hours. The carb cycling diet takes a great commitment, but if done properly, the results can be amazing.

As with any diet, you need to make sure you will be able to stick to it for it to be effective. For many people, crab cycling is too time consuming and they prefer diet plans that set meal plans for them. The benefit of carb cycling is that you can eat anything as long is it is on the right day. The truth is all diets will have restrictions; you just need to make sure your body can handle whatever diet you are on.

CARB CYCLE HISTORY

In the seventies and eighties there was a "high-carb mania" where the popular diets of the day recommended eating large amounts of carbohydrates. Then, in the nineties through today, the opposite became popular. Nowadays people everywhere seem to be avoiding carbs. In fact, this "low-carb mania" has swept the whole world and created legions of low-carb fanatics. Still, most people are confused and have no clue how the human body actually uses carbs and how a certain carb lifestyle can either help you lose weight or totally destroy any weight loss results. Today, there are more diets, exercise books, videos, classes, trainers, fitness experts, and information available than ever before. However, at the same time, the majority of people are frustrated and still out of shape. In fact overweight and obesity are taking over the world. Why is this? The reason is that no fitness system on the market really puts into consideration how the human body is created to function. Most diets eventually end up slowing down the metabolism, and therefore any weight loss effort is put to a halt due to no energy or loss of motivation. To Summarize: constant low-carb or constant high or moderate-carb diets are just NOT the solution to fight obesity and get and stay lean and healthy!

Carb Cycle 1: It was also in the nineties when Franco Carlotto, the creator of Carb Cycle, developed a way of eating carbs right that made him win six Mr. World Fitness Titles as well as helping people from all over the world and all walks of life to achieve and maintain a lean, fit, and healthy body. Now, for the first time ever, he's ready to share his method with the whole world and you publicly. His goal was to develop a diet approach for everybody that offers results both, in the short-term and long-term.

Franco realized over 20 years ago that the solution to eating right today, lies in our past, evolving back to the same way our ancestors continuously loaded and depleted their carb storage. Since our bodies didn't change since then, this is still the key to ultimate weight control in the 21st Century: the human body's own carb storage system! Franco's Carb Cycle is the only fitness and nutrition program that works with that natural carb storage system - something most people don't even know they have - in this intended and correct way.

Carb Cycle 2: Franco's Carb Cycle regulates the body's natural storage mechanism for carbs by alternating between normal-carb and low-carb days in an ongoing cycle which repeats itself twice every week. It is the only Method that first depletes and then loads the body's carb storage in an appropriate, most efficient, and simple to execute cycle. Best of all, at any given point, you never have to totally sacrifice your carbs, but just slightly increase and lower certain carbs on certain days of the week in a very easy to manage manner. Although there are many fine-tuning options and Franco's System offers an "Advanced Carb Cycle" section, once you implement his Basic Carb Cycle knowledge into your diet, it literally forces your body to burn it's fat depots down to a minimum while - contrary to most other diet and fitness systems - giving you energy and speeding up your metabolism, both, in the short-term and long-term! It further allows you to eat all kind of foods and meals - including carbs - guilt-free on a regular basis without having to deprive your body's metabolism of much-needed energy to function properly.

Carb Cycle 3 Franco Carlotto's Carb Cycle Method is not just another diet or fitness hype. It is a fitness guide to life. Based on his 27 years of experience, he's explaining what the Carb Cycle is, how it evolved, and how it works. Most importantly he outlays exactly how to implement the Carb Cycle right away into your own, individual lifestyle.

Franco guides you one-on-one with food plans, recipes, food choices, and many more tips and tricks all around carbs and fitness. Most importantly, he lays out the 3 Carb.

Cycle Stages to choose from for any fitness level: from 1) Starter to 2) Intermediate to 3) Advanced. Thereafter, with Stage 4 - Carb Cycle for Life - he will show you how to maintain your newfound body for good.

EXAMPLE CARB CYCLING MENU

Here are three sample meal plans for low-, moderate- and high-carb days.

HIGH-CARB DAY

* Breakfast: 3 boiled eggs, 3 slices Ezekiel (or 7 seed/grain) bread, tomatoes, mushrooms and a side bowl of mixed fruit (60 g carbs).

* Lunch: 6 oz sweet potato, 6 oz lean meat or fish, mixed vegetables (45 g carbs).

* Pre-Workout: 1 serving oatmeal, almond milk, 1 cup berries, 1 scoop whey protein (50 g carbs).

* Dinner: 1 serving wholemeal rice, 6 oz lean chicken, homemade tomato sauce, 1 serving kidney beans, mixed vegetables (70 g carbs).

MODERATE-CARB DAY

* Breakfast: Grass-fed high-protein yogurt, 1 cup mixed berries, stevia, 1 spoon seed mix (25 g carbs).

* Lunch: 6 oz chicken salad with 4 oz diced potatoes (25 g carbs).

* Pre-Workout: 1 banana with whey protein shake (30 g carbs).

* Dinner: 1 serving sweet potato fries, 6 oz lean beef, homemade tomato sauce, 1 serving kidney beans, mixed vegetables (40 g carbs).

LOW-CARB DAY

* Breakfast: 3 eggs with 3 slices bacon and mixed vegetables (10 g carbs).

* Lunch: 6 oz salmon salad with 1 spoon olive oil (10 g carbs).

* Snack: 1 oz mixed nuts with 1 serving turkey slices (10 g carbs).

* Dinner: 6 oz steak, half avocado, mixed vegetables (16 g carbs).

RECOMMENDED CARBOHYDRATE FOOD SOURCES

Some carbohydrates should be avoided, except on special occasions or for the occasional treat.

In contrast, there are plenty of healthy carb sources that are tasty and packed full of beneficial fiber, vitamins and minerals.

When planning your high-carb days, do not use it as an excuse for an all-out pop-tart binge. Instead, focus on these healthier carb choices.

RECOMMENDED "GOOD" CARBS:

* Whole Grains: Unmodified grains are perfectly healthy and linked with many health benefits. Sources include: brown rice, oats and quinoa.

* Vegetables: Every vegetable has a different vitamin and mineral content, eat a variety of colors to get a good balance.

* Unprocessed Fruits: As with vegetables, every fruit is unique, especially berries with their high antioxidant content and low glycemic load.

* Legumes: A great choice of slow digesting carbohydrates, which are full of fiber and minerals. Just make sure you prepare them properly.

* Tubers: Potatoes, sweet potatoes, etc.

CARB CYCLING - IS IT NECESSARY?

When you are trying to lose weight, its often a good idea to control your carb intake. Not because carbs are bad, but because carbs (like pasta and rice) are tasty and easily available. We often tend to overeat them and pack on the calories. Personally, I have had great success by controlling my carb intake for dinners. You are more likely to overeat carbs during dinner than any other meal. Replacing a regular high carb dinner with a salad will save you hundreds of calories daily!!!

However, if your lower caloric intake continues for a long time, your body will adapt to it by lowering your metabolism. For e.g. If your body required 2500 daily calories to maintain weight and you only ate 2000 calories, you body would initially lose a pound every week. Do this long enough and your body will lower your daily maintenance level to match 2000 calories.

What happens then? You stop losing weight!!!!

So the logic goes you should vary your calorie consumption to keep the body from adapting to a lower calorie diet. How do you do it? You cycle your carb/ calorie intake to increase or decrease the amount of calories you consume. Some people cycle daily, others cycle every 3-4 days.

There are many variations of carb cycling or calorie cycling. For e.g. You eat salad for dinner 3 days in a row. Then on the fourth day you have a serving of pasta or rice with your dinner. Or you might add some dessert to your dinner. This will raise the calorie intake by 400-500 calories for that day and then you repeat the cycle. This "peak" in calories keeps the body from slowing down the metabolism.

SHOULD YOU USE CARB CYCLING TO LOSE WEIGHT?

Well the answer is not as simple. It all depends on how much weight you have to lose and how intensely you have been exercising.

Ignore carb cycling if you...

...have more than 20 pounds to lose, you can focus on creating calorie deficit on a weekly basis through nutrition and exercise.

...are successfully losing weight every week with your current diet and exercise plan. Don't fix what isn't broken.

You should use carb cycling if you...

...have less than 20 pounds to lose. The leaner and fitter you are, the more your body will resist losing weight. So you will need to trick your body into shedding those last few pounds.

...Have stopped losing weight. If you are already eating smaller portions, then cutting calories further can backfire. You could try exercising more, but at some point that won't be enough.

CARB CYCLING MEAL PLAN - LEARN THE IMPORTANCE OF PROTEIN IN THE CARB CYCLING DIET

There are many carb cycling meal plans out there, however, not all of them are going to have the foods that you like on them. So, maybe it's time to create one of your own.

Here, I will show you what types of foods, and why they should be going into your meal plans.

The carb cycling meal plans are best done on a 6 meal a day plan, this way you will have enough food to fuel you, and keep your metabolism up, which is very important in this diet.

There are 3 basic days in the carb cycling diet:

- High Carb Day

- Low Carb Day

- No Carb Day

On the high carb day, you are going to have 4 meals out of 6 which will contain as many carbs as you want. Just remember to mix it up with some lean proteins such as:

- white chicken/turkey meat

- tuna fish (canned)

- protein shakes with at least 40 - 50g of protein in them. Remember, you will want to go 1g / 1 lbs of body weight when you consume protein. This will help maintain your muscle definition.

- cottage cheese

- and egg whites.

Those are the best proteins you can consume during your run of the carb cycling diet.

On the low carb day, you cut back on the carbs to only a limited 3 meals with any carbs at all. All others will have none, just lots of lean proteins, and veggies. Your proteins are very important on this day, as they will be a major part of your diet, so don't skimp out.

On the no carb day you are going to have NO to LITTLE carb intake at all. Most of the carbs will come from the veggies, or protein that you will eat through out the day.

As you can see through out those 3 basic cycle days, you have to keep up your protein intake. This is what feeds your muscles, without it, you lose them, and your metabolism drops like a rock. Since keeping your metabolism up through out the diet is the key to making it work then that would mean that eating your proper intake of protein is the key to the whole thing.

Without the proper protein intake at 1g / 1 lbs of body weight, the carb cycling meal plan will be null and void. Because without it, there is no metabolism, because there is no muscle to start it up. So while on the carb cycling diet, please keep up the required intake of protein, this way, you will actually stand a chance in reaching your goal of a nicely defined body.

CARB CYCLING RECIPES

On the surface, the carb cycle diet couldn't be more simple. On days you work out the most, you eat a lot of healthy carbs, like whole grains or legumes. On less-intense training days, you limit carbs and focus on eating protein-rich foods and low-carb veggies. The carb-heavy days give you the energy you need to fuel your workouts, adherents say, while the low-carb days help you lose weight.

"Eating healthy carbs on certain days keeps your metabolism revved up, and sticking to mostly protein and vegetables on days in between keeps insulin low enough that you can burn fat without losing muscle," Shelby Starnes, a competitive bodybuilder and carb cycling expert, told Daily Burn.

Carb cycling might not seem terribly complex, especially compared to some diet plans, but it still requires work if you're going to stick to it, especially over the long term. Boredom can easily set in if you always end up cooking a plain chicken breast and steamed broccoli for dinner on your low-carb days.

To help you reach your fitness goals and shed those extra pounds, I have listed out some creative low-carb recipes that will help you stick to your carb cycle diet.

10 BREAKFAST CARB CYCLING RECIPES

1. BALSAMIC BRUSSELS SPROUTS WITH ALMOND-ENCRUSTED SEARED TUNA

An almond coating gives low-fat, high-protein tuna steaks some extra crunch in this quick-cooking dinner recipe.

For your vegetable side, Brussels sprouts are slowly cooked in coconut oil and balsamic vinegar until tender.

INGREDIENTS:

For the Brussels sprouts:

- 1½ pounds Brussels sprouts, trimmed and split

- ¼ cup coconut oil

- 1 tablespoon thick balsamic vinegar

- Sea salt and black pepper to taste

For the tuna:

- 3 tuna steaks

- Crushed almonds

- Sea salt to taste

- Pepper to taste

- 2 tablespoons coconut oil

DIRECTIONS:

1. To prepare Brussels sprouts, add coconut oil to a saucepan and turn heat to medium-high. When the oil melts, add the Brussels sprouts, salt, and pepper, then mix.

2. Cover, reduce heat to low, and let cook for 15 minutes.

3. Add the balsamic vinegar to the pan and stir. Cover and cook on low for 10 more minutes, until Brussels sprouts are tender.

4. To make the tuna, crush the almonds using a food processor or rolling pin. Salt and pepper the tuna steaks. Press each tuna steak into the crushed almonds to coat, then flip and repeat on the other side.

5. In a large frying pan, heat the coconut oil until melted and clear. Place tuna steaks in the pan and sear for 2 minutes. Flip and continue to cook for another 2 minutes.

6. Remove the steaks from the pan and slice into strips. Serve with the Brussels sprouts.

2. ZUPPA TOSCANA

This spin on a traditional Tuscan soup replaces potato with cauliflower for a dish that retains its rich flavor without piling on the carbs. Make a batch on Sunday and you'll have enough for a week's work of breakfast.

INGREDIENTS:

- 2 cups chicken stock
- 1 quart water
- 1 pound Italian sausage, ground
- 3 cups kale, chopped
- 2 cups cauliflower, riced
- 2 cloves garlic, chopped
- ½ cup onion, diced
- 1 tablespoon heavy whipping cream
- 1 teaspoon crushed red pepper
- ¼ cup butter
- Salt and pepper to taste
- Fresh-grated Parmesan for serving (optional)

DIRECTIONS:

1. Brown the sausage, onion, and garlic in a large saucepan. After the meat is fully cooked and the onions are soft and translucent, use a little of the chicken stock to the pan, scraping up any bits that are stuck to the bottom of the pan.

2. Add the water, rest of the stock, crushed red pepper, salt, and pepper to

the pan. Let simmer for about 30 minutes.

3. Add the butter, kale, and cauliflower. Cook for about 15 minutes, until vegetables are tender. Just before serving, stir in 1 tablespoon of heavy whipping cream. Garnish with fresh-grated Parmesan if you like.

3. LOW-CARB BEEF AND BROCCOLI STIR FRY

When served sans rice, a beef and broccoli stir fry is the perfect option for a quick, low-carb dinner. Unfortunately, many recipes call for coating your meat and veggies in a sweet sauce made thickened with flour or cornstarch – not exactly what you want on a low-carb day.

INGREDIENTS:

- 1 tablespoon canola oil
- 2 cups broccoli, blanched
- ½ cup thinly sliced carrot
- ½ cup onion, cut into wedges
- 6 ounces sirloin steak, boneless and cut into strips
- 1½ tablespoons chicken broth
- 1 tablespoon low-sodium soy sauce
- ½ teaspoon guar gum or cornstarch
- ¼ teaspoon Splenda sugar substitute
- 1/8 teaspoon salt (optional)

DIRECTIONS:

1. Heat the oil in a large skillet. Add the broccoli, carrot, and onion and cook, stirring frequently, until the vegetables are tender-crisp. Stir in the beef and cook until it reaches desired doneness.

2. Stir together the chicken broth, soy sauce, guar gum, Splenda, and salt in a small bowl. Add to the beef and vegetables and cook, stirring constantly until the sauce thickens, about 2 to 3 minutes.

4. FLANK STEAK SALAD WITH CHIMICHURRI DRESSING

A grilled steak is served on a bed of healthy green and dressed with a delicious chimichurri sauce in this easy-to-make main dish salad.

- 1 large bunch fresh Italian parsley

- 2 tablespoons fresh oregano leaves

- 3 garlic cloves, peeled

- ½ cup olive oil

- ¼ cup red wine vinegar

- 1 teaspoon chipotle hot pepper sauce

- 1½ pounds flank steak

- 8 ounces mixed baby greens

- 12-ounce container marinated small fresh mozzarella balls, drained

DIRECTIONS:

1. Prepare barbecue (medium-high heat). Combine parsley (with stems), oregano, and garlic in processor; blend 10 seconds. Add ½ cup oil, vinegar, and hot pepper sauce; blend until almost smooth. Season dressing to taste with salt and pepper.

2. Brush grill rack with oil. Sprinkle steak on both sides with salt and pepper. Grill steak to desired doneness, about 5 minutes per side for medium-rare. Transfer steak to work surface; let rest 5 minutes.

3. Meanwhile, toss greens in large bowl with some dressing. Transfer to large platter. Sprinkle mozzarella over.

4. Thinly slice steak across grain on slight diagonal. Arrange steak atop greens. Drizzle with remaining dressing.

5. SEARED SCALLOPS AND WILTED GREENS

Hearty scallops are seared in butter and oil and then served on a bed of shallots and wilted greens cooked with thick-cut bacon in this recipe from A Spicy Perspective. Best of all, you can prepare this flavorful and filling dish in under 30 minutes.

INGREDIENTS:

- 3 slices of thick-cut bacon, cut into pieces
- 2 shallots, sliced thin
- 2 to 3 cloves garlic, minced
- 2 bunches of kale (or substitute chard or beet greens)
- 1 tablespoon soy sauce
- 1 tablespoon red wine vinegar
- Salt
- Pepper
- 12 large sea scallops
- 2 tablespoons olive oil
- 1 tablespoon butter

DIRECTIONS:

1. Slice kale leaves into large strips and the stems into thin pieces. Set aside.

2. Heat a large, high-sided pan over medium-high heat. Add the bacon and cook for 3 to 4 minutes. Add the shallots and continue to cook for another 3 to 4 minutes. Add the garlic and kale stems to the pan and cook for 4 to 5 minutes. Then, add the kale leaves and toss until wilted.

3. Add the soy sauce, vinegar, and pepper to the kale and bacon mixture. Set aside and keep warm.

4. Heat a cast-iron skillet over high heat. Dry the scallops, then season with salt and pepper. Add olive oil to the pan and swirl to coat. When the oil begins to smoke, add the scallops and cook for 1 to 2 minutes.

5. Flip the scallops and add the butter to the pan. Continue to cook for another 1 to 2 minutes. Serve over the warm kale and bacon.

6. FRIED EGGS WITH PROSCIUTTO AND ASPARAGUS

A fried egg with prosciutto and asparagus is perfect for either a quick lunch or a simple dinner. Blanching the asparagus for just a few minutes ensures that your vegetables are tender enough to eat but not limp and soggy.

INGREDIENTS:

- 1 pound (16 spears) asparagus
- Salt
- Freshly ground black pepper
- 1 tablespoon unsalted butter, melted
- 4 large eggs
- ¼ pound thinly sliced prosciutto
- 2 tablespoons freshly grated Parmesan cheese
- 1 tablespoon coarsely chopped flat-leaf parsley

DIRECTIONS:

1. Snap off and discard tough ends of asparagus. Bring a large sauté pan of salted water to a boil. Cook asparagus until just tender but still dark green, 4 to 5 minutes. Transfer to a clean kitchen towel; fold over. Set aside.

2. Heat half of the butter in a large nonstick skillet over medium-low heat. Break eggs into skillet. Season with salt and pepper, and cook, covered, until set, about 4 minutes.

3. Place several slices of prosciutto on each of four plates; arrange 4 spears asparagus on each. Brush with the remaining melted butter. Carefully place fried eggs on top, sprinkle with Parmesan and parsley, and serve.

7. 5-MINUTE SPICY ASIAN CHICKEN SALAD

On the surface, the carb cycle diet couldn't be more simple. On days you work out the most, you eat a lot of healthy carbs, like whole grains or legumes. On less-intense training days, you limit carbs and focus on eating protein-rich foods and low-carb veggies. The carb-heavy days give you the energy you need to fuel your workouts, adherents say, while the low-carb days help you lose weight.

"Eating healthy carbs on certain days keeps your metabolism revved up, and sticking to mostly protein and vegetables on days in between keeps insulin low enough that you can burn fat without losing muscle," Shelby Starnes, a competitive bodybuilder and carb cycling expert, told Daily Burn.

Carb cycling might not seem terribly complex, especially compared to some diet plans, but it still requires work if you're going to stick to it, especially over the long term.

Boredom can easily set in if you always end up cooking a plain chicken breast and steamed broccoli for dinner on your low-carb days.

To help you reach your fitness goals and shed those extra pounds, here are seven creative low-carb recipes that will help you stick to your carb cycle diet.

8. BALSAMIC BRUSSELS SPROUTS

SHOPPING LIST:

ALL ORGANIC INGREDIENTS

- 1 1/2 pounds Brussels sprouts, trimmed and split

- 1/4 cup coconut oil

- 1 tablespoon thick balsamic vinegar

- Sea salt and black pepper to taste

DIRECTIONS:

1. Put saucepan on medium high, and add coconut oil to pan.

2. When oil is melted, add Brussel sprouts, salt and pepper, and mix with a spoon.

3. Cover and turn down to low.

4. 15 minutes later, add balsamic vinegar and mix with spoon. Re-cover on low heat for ten more minutes.

5. Brussel sprouts are fork tender when ready

9. COCONUT OIL FRENCH FRIES:

SHOPPING LIST:

ALL ORGANIC INGREDIENTS

- 3 Red or sweet potatoes (I generally do one potato per person), sliced with a food slicer wavy (or cut thin with a sharp knife)

- 3 cups coconut oil

- Sea salt and pepper to taste

DIRECTIONS:

1. Wash potatoes and slice them (I used my Nutrichef food slicer on setting one, you can use a food slicer or a sharp knife to cut chips).

2. Soak in water for 20 minutes (This step is important. My French fries always taste better because of this!)

3. Melt coconut oil in deep-frying pan. I used my Nutrichef electric skillet.

4. When fully melted, add potatoes into oil and cook until light golden brown.

5. When you remove the fries, lay them on a paper towel and salt to taste! They are so delicious, the kids always get them before they make it to the table.

10. ALMOND ENCRUSTED SEARED TUNA:

SHOPPING LIST:

ALL ORGANIC INGREDIENTS

- 3 tuna steaks

- Crusted almonds

- Sea salt and pepper to taste

- 2 tablespoons coconut oil

DIRECTIONS:

1. Crush almonds. (You can crush them extra fine or leave them chunky like I did. I like the texture that way.)

2. Salt and pepper tuna steaks to taste.

3. Press tuna steaks into the almonds on both sides.

4. Heat coconut oil in a large frying pan on medium heat until clear

5. Add tuna steaks and sear on each side for two minutes. Remove and slice steaks into strips.

10 LUNCH CARB CYCLING RECIPES

1. HONEY SOY STRAWBERRY VINAIGRETTE SAUCE:

SHOPPING LIST:

ALL ORGANIC INGREDIENTS

- 1 tablespoon raw local honey

- 2 tablespoons of strawberry vinaigrette

- 1 tablespoon soy sauce

Directions:

1. Mix ingredients together and serve.

2. ORECCHIETTE WITH SAUSAGE AND BROCCOLI

Servings: 4-6

INGREDIENTS

- 1 pound orecchiette

- 5 tablespoons extra virgin olive oil, divided

- 1 pound sweet Italian sausage, removed from casings

- 3 garlic cloves, minced

- 1 cup chicken broth

- 1 pound broccoli florets

- 1/2 teaspoon salt

- 1/4 teaspoon red pepper flakes

- 3 tablespoons unsalted butter

- 1/2 cup freshly grated Pecorino Romano

INSTRUCTIONS

1. Bring a large pot of salted water to a boil. Add the orecchiette and cook according to package instructions.

2. Meanwhile, in a large skillet, heat 1 tablespoon of the olive oil over medium high heat. Crumble the sausage into the skillet and cook, breaking apart with a spoon, until lightly browned, 5-6 minutes. Reduce the heat to medium and add the garlic; cook for 1 minute more.

3. Add the remaining 4 tablespoons of olive oil, chicken broth, broccoli, salt and red pepper flakes. Cook, stirring frequently and scraping the bottom of the pan to release the flavorful brown bits, until the broccoli is tender-crisp, 3-4 minutes. Stir in the butter until melted and simmer for a

few minutes to reduce and concentrate the sauce.

4. Drain the pasta well and add to the sausage and broccoli mixture. Toss to blend. Add half of the grated cheese taste and stir until the cheese is melted. Taste and adjust seasoning. Transfer to a serving platter or individual bowls and sprinkle with the rest of the grated cheese.

3. LEMON-TAHINI CUCUMBER NOODLES WITH SHRIMP

INGREDIENTS

FOR THE SALAD:

- 1 large English/seedless cucumber
- 2 roma tomatoes, seeded and diced
- 3 tablespoons minced mint
- 2 tablespoons minced parsley
- ? cup diced red onion
- ? cup pitted and halved kalamata olives
- ½ teaspoon sumac or paprika

FOR THE SHRIMP:

- 8 large or 12 small shrimp, defrosted, peeled, deveined
- 2 teaspoons extra virgin olive oil
- ½ teaspoon garlic powder (or to taste)
- salt and pepper

FOR THE DRESSING:

- 2 tablespoons tahini
- 2 tablespoons freshly squeezed lemon juice
- 1 teaspoon honey
- 1 small garlic clove, minced
- 2 tablespoons water, to thin

- salt & pepper, to taste

INSTRUCTIONS

1. Place all of the ingredients for the dressing into a food processor and pulse until creamy. Taste and adjust to your preference, if needed. Set aside.

2. Slice the cucumber halfway lengthwise and then spiralize it. Pat the noodles dry with paper towels and then place in a large mixing bowl, along with the tomato, mint, parsley and onion. Set aside.

3. Place a medium skillet over medium-high heat and add in the oil. Once oil heats, add in the shrimp and season with salt, pepper and garlic powder. Cook for 2 minutes, flip over and cook another 2 minutes or until shrimp are opaque and cooked through.

4. Transfer the cucumber mixture to a plate, top with dressing and then shrimp. Sprinkle over with sumac (or paprika) and enjoy.

4. SPANISH CAULIFLOWER 'RICE'

Cauliflower is perhaps one of the most versatile vegetables. You can roast it, make a pizza, make a sauce, make wings, and make bites of all other varieties. Best of all, you can make cauliflower rice, which is a million more times filling than the standard rice as it packs more fiber, and more nutrients to boot! This Spanish-inspired cauliflower rice dish is packed with flavor, heat, and the refreshing bite of lime and cilantro.

INGREDIENTS

- 1 large head cauliflower, shredded or finely ground
- 1/2 red onion, shredded or diced
- 2 cloves garlic, shredded or minced
- 1 tablespoon olive oil
- 2 tablespoons adobo sauce
- 1/2 cup salsa
- 3/4 cup black beans, rinsed
- 1 jalapeño or serrano chili, halved (optional), or substitute 1 small can of diced green chilis
- 1 teaspoon salt, or more to taste
- 1 lime
- 2 sprigs of cilantro
- 1 avocado

INSTRUCTIONS:

Step 1: Shred cauliflower in a food processor by pulsing until finely ground into pieces slightly larger than cooked rice. Dice onion, jalapeño, and mince garlic.

Step 2: Heat a large sauté pan or skillet over medium heat, add olive oil, garlic, jalapeño, chili powder, and salt. Cook for a minute to flavor the oil. Increase the heat to high, add onion, and cook until translucent. Then add black beans and cook for a few minutes before adding adobo sauce, lime juice, and lastly cauliflower.

Step 3: Cook for 6-8 minutes, stirring often, until the moisture is evaporated and the cauliflower is light and fluffy. Strain if needed. Top with lime juice, avocado, and cilantro.

5. BEET AND GOAT CHEESE PIZZA WITH CAULIFLOWER CRUST

Low carb and gluten free has never looked so pretty and inventive. A cauliflower crust is topped with pureed beets, goat cheese, candied walnuts, and fresh arugula.

Serves: 2-3

Ingredients:

CAULIFLOWER CRUST

- 1/2 large head cauliflower

- 1 egg, lightly beaten

- 2 oz. goat cheese, crumbled

- 1 Tbsp fresh minced oregano (or 1 tsp dried)

- 1 Tbsp minced garlic (about 2 cloves)

- Salt and pepper, to taste

BEET SAUCE

- 1 (15 oz.) can whole beets, rinsed and drained

- 2 Tbsp extra virgin olive oil

- 1 Tbsp balsamic vinegar

- 1/2 Tbsp minced garlic (about 1 clove)

- 1/2 tsp crushed red pepper (optional)

- Salt and pepper to taste

TOPPINGS

- 1 cup walnuts

- 2 Tbsp brown sugar

- 1 Tbsp honey

- Pinch Salt

- 4 oz. goat cheese, crumbled

- 2 handfuls fresh baby arugula

DIRECTIONS:

1. Preheat oven to 450 degrees. Generously coat a cookie sheet or pizza pan with nonstick spray, set aside.

2. Use a cheese grater or food processor to shred the cauliflower into small crumbles (NOT puree). You should have 2 cups, if not shred more. Place cauliflower in a large microwave-safe bowl and microwave for 8 minutes. Allow to cool, then squeeze out excess liquid using a colander and paper towels.

3. Return cauliflower to the large bowl. Add remaining crust ingredients and stir until blended. Dump the mixture onto the prepared pan and pat into about a 12-inch circle. Spray crust lightly with nonstick spray and bake for 15-20 minutes, or until golden.

4. While the crust bakes, prepare the beet sauce. Add beets to a food processor (or blender) and pulse until finely chopped. Add olive oil, balsamic vinegar, garlic, and red pepper (if using). Pulse until smooth. Season with salt and pepper to taste. Set aside and prepare the candied walnuts.

5. In a small skillet over medium heat combine the walnuts, brown sugar, and honey. Cook until the sugar melts and forms a thick syrup, stirring constantly, about 3-4 minutes. Immediately pour onto a parchment or silicone-lined baking sheet. Spread out into a single layer and allow to cool.

6. When the crust is cooked and golden, remove from oven. Spread beet sauce over the pre-baked crust and sprinkle with goat cheese. Bake for another 5-10 minutes or until the cheese is soft and bubbly.

7. Sprinkle with candied walnuts and fresh arugula. Cut into 6 slices and serve immediately.

6. CAPRESE GRILLED FILET MIGNON

Serves: 4-6

Adjust Servings

Add summer flair to grilled steak by topping those filets with the classic salad of tomatoes, fresh mozzarella, and basil.

INGREDIENTS

- four 6-8 oz filets
- kosher salt and freshly ground pepper
- olive oil
- 1-2 roma tomatoes, sliced about 1/4 inch thick (you'll need eight slices)
- About 4 oz fresh mozzarella, cut into four slices
- About eight fresh basil leaves
- Reduced balsamic vinegar

INSTRUCTIONS

1. Season filets with salt and pepper and lightly brush with olive oil

2. Heat grill to high. Place steaks on grill, reduce heat to medium. Cover

and cook for 5 minutes.

3. Flip and cook for an additional 5 minutes.

4. Reduce to low, top with one tomato slice, one basil leaf, one slice mozzarella, another basil leaf, and another slice of tomato.

5. Close the cover and grill for another 3-5 minutes or to desired doneness.

6. Remove to a platter, let rest for at least 5 minutes, drizzle with olive oil and reduced balsamic vinegar before serving.

7.CHIPOTLE CHICKEN SALAD STUFFED AVOCADOS

Chipotle Chicken Salad Stuffed Avocados are low-carb recipe full of fresh vegetables and flavor from a spicy chipotle sauce for a light and healthy packed lunch idea!

Prep Time: 10 mins

Total Time: 10 mins

Recipe type: Lunch

Serves: 4

INGREDIENTS

- 1 c. cooked chicken, cubed
- ? c. onions, diced
- ¼ c. bell pepper, diced
- ? c. tomatoes, chopped
- ? c. chipotle sauce (1/3 of sauce)
- 2 avocados
- chipotle lime sauce
- ? c. non-fat plain greek yogurt
- ¼ c. mayo
- 1 Tbsp lime juice
- 1 chipotle pepper in adobe

- 1 Tbsp adobe sauce

- ½ tsp salt

- 1 tsp garlic, finely chopped

- 1 tsp cumin

INSTRUCTIONS

1. Toss all of the chicken salad ingredients in a small bowl until all of the chicken and vegetables are well coated with the chipotle sauce.

2. Halve and remove the seeds from the avocados. Slice a small piece off the bottom of each half so the avocado sits flat.

3. Spoon the chicken salad mixture into each avocado half and serve immediately.

8. PALEO SAVORY ITALIAN TART

Prep Time: 1 hour

Cook Time: 35-40min

Servings: 5

INGREDIENTS

For the Crust:

- 1 3/4 cups raw cashews
- 1/4 cup potato starch
- 2 teaspoons organic Italian seasoning
- 1 teaspoon sea salt
- 1 egg white
- 1-3 tablespoons unsweetened almond milk

FOR THE PESTO FILLING:

- 2 cups basil leaves
- 1/2 cup oregano leaves
- 1/4 cup olive oil
- 3 garlic cloves
- 1 teaspoons sea salt
- 1/2 teaspoon freshly ground pepper
- 1/4 cup pine nuts

- 1-2 tablespoons fresh lemon juice

FOR THE TURKEY MEAT:

- 1/2 pound ground turkey (lean, not fat free...see note)
- 1/2 teaspoon organic garlic powder
- 1/2 teaspoon smoked paprika
- 1/2 teaspoon organic cumin
- 2 teaspoon organic Italian seasoning
- 1 teaspoon sea salt

FOR THE VEGGIES ON TOP:

- 1/2 cup tomatoes (sliced)
- 1/2 cup zucchinis (sliced)
- 1/2 cup purple onions (sliced)

EXTRAS FOR DRIZZLING:

- sea salt
- balsamic vinegar
- parmesan cheese (optional)
- coconut oil spray

INSTRUCTIONS:

For the Crust:

1. Preheat the oven to 350 degrees F.

2. Combine all of the ingredients for the crust in your food processor, except the almond milk.

3. Run it on high, until the cashews are broken into a fine flour and everything is well incorporated.

4. Add the almond milk, one tablespoon at a time. Run the processor after each tablespoon. Keep adding until the mixture starts to clump together, as in the picture.

5. Grease a large rectangular tart pan with coconut oil spray, then press the pie dough into it. Make sure to make the dough as flat and even as possible, pushing it up the sides of the pan, as well.

6. Precook the crust for 12 minutes, then set it aside until you are ready to fill it. You can prep the fillings while it bakes.For the Pesto:

7. Combine all of the ingredients for your pesto in a food processor and run it on high until the pesto is smooth. Pesto will be the first layer in your crust.For the Turkey:

8. Heat your pan over medium heat, then add all of the ingredients. Use a spatula to break up the meat and mix everything well. Cook until the meat is completely cooked through.Finishing Up:

9. Make sure all of your veggies are sliced and ready to layer, and that your oven is still heated. It's best to make your veggie slices roughly the same size and thickness.

10. Layer the ingredients into your pie crust, starting with the pesto. After the pesto comes the meat, and after the meat comes the vegetables.

11. Sprinkle the top of your tart with sea salt, parmesan cheese (if desired), and balsamic vinegar, then spray it liberally with the coconut oil spray. Use a generous amount of balsamic vinegar…it adds a ton of flavor to this dish!!!

12. Bake the tart until the veggies are wilting and starting to brown a little. 25-30 minutes should do it! Serve warm, with extra balsamic vinegar and sea salt. Enjoy!

9. MISO-TAHINI TURMERIC DRESSING

Miso is a fermented soybean paste that is often used in recipes to give the meal a savory, almost meaty flavor (umami). Miso paste can be used in soups, sauces, or marinades, as well as in dressing, like this recipe. Because it is fermented, miso paste contains probiotics, which are good bacteria that aid in regular digestion, bowel movements, and a strong immune system.

Prep Time: 5 minutes

Cook Time: 0 minutes

Servings: 2

INGREDIENTS:

- 1 teaspoon white miso paste (use chickpea miso for a soy-free option)
- 3 tablespoon warm (not boiling water, divided)
- 1/4 cup tahini
- 1/4 teaspoon turmeric (optional)
- black pepper to taste (optional)

INSTRUCTIONS

1. Dissolve miso in 1 tablespoon warm water until there are no clumps.

2. Add tahini, stirring until well combined, then add 1 tablespoon of room temp water at a time until you reach your desired consistency.

3. Add turmeric and black pepper and stir until combined.

*To thicken, add less water. For a salad dressing, add a little more water.

Note: This sauce will thicken when kept in the fridge. Just add 1 teaspoon of water at a time if it needs thinning when you take it out.

NUTRITION INFORMATION:

Per Serving: **Calories**: 205; **Total Fat**: 18g; **Saturated Fat**: 3g; **Monounsaturated Fat**: 0g; **Polyunsaturated Fat**: 0g; **Cholesterol**: 0mg; **Sodium**: 205mg; **Potassium**: 124mg;

Carbohydrate: 4g; Fiber: 1g; Sugar: 0g; Protein: 5g

Nutrition Bonus: Iron: 9%

10. BLT CHOPPED SALAD WITH CORN, FETA + AVOCADO

Yield: serves 2

Total Time: 25 minutes

INGREDIENTS:

- 2 cups butter lettuce, chopped
- 2 cups fresh arugula, chopped
- 1 pint grape tomatos, quartered
- 4 slices thick-cut bacon, fried and crumbled
- 1 cup sweet corn
- 1 avocado, chopped
- 4 ounces feta, crumbled
- 1 1/2 tablespoons olive oil
- 1 lime, juiced
- 1/4 teaspoon salt
- 1/4 teaspoon pepper

DIRECTIONS:

1. As a note, to chop my lettuce I like to lay it out on a big cutting board and just continuously run my knife through it (in all different directions) until it's chopped as much as I like.

2. In a large bowl, combine lettuce, arugula, tomatoes, corn and avocado. Add in salt, pepper, olive oil and lime juice then toss well to coat. Fold in bacon and feta then divide evenly amount 2 plates. Serve!

10 DINNER CARB CYLCING RECIPES

1. CREAMY GARLIC SPAGHETTI SQUASH CASSEROLE (PALEO, GLUTEN-FREE, AND DAIRY-FREE)

This creamy garlic spaghetti squash casserole is so saucy and delicious! Do you long for a creamy, dairy-free sauce packed with garlicky goodness? Well, look no more! Plus, this dish is made with spaghetti squash, which is a much healthier casserole option. Go ahead, get your squash on, and make a big old pan of this filling and flavorful casserole!

Prep Time: 5 minutes

Cook Time: 55 minutes

Servings: 6

Ingredients

- 1 medium spaghetti squash

- 4 cups broccoli florets

- 1 pound sausage (spicy Italian or Chorizo are excellent choices)

- 2 cups mushrooms – diced

- 2 tablespoons minced garlic

- 16 ounces coconut milk

- 1/4 cup arrowroot flour

- Salt and pepper

INSTRUCTIONS

1. Preheat oven to 425 degrees Fahrenheit.

2. Slice the spaghetti squash lengthwise and scoop out the seeds. Place the two halves face-down on a baking sheet and place in the oven to bake for 30 minutes.

3. While the squash is cooking, get the sausage going. Heat a large pan over medium heat and add in the sausage.

4. Break it into pieces with a spatula and cook, stirring occasionally, until browned and cooked through, about 8 minutes. Remove from pan and set aside. Reserve at least 1 tbsp of fat in the pan for the sauce you'll make later.

5. Remove squash from oven after 30 minutes and set aside to cool. Keep the oven on at 425 degrees.

6. While the squash is cooling, prepare the creamy garlic sauce. Heat the same pan you cooked the sausage in over medium heat. Once hot, add mushrooms and cook until they begin to soften, about 2 minutes. Add in the arrowroot flour and crushed garlic and stir around to mix well with the mushrooms, about 1-2 minutes.

7. Next, add in coconut milk, stirring constantly for 2 minutes. Be sure to mix well to dissolve all of the flour into the milk (you don't want any flour clumps). Use a whisk to mix if needed. The sauce will bubble and thicken, keep stirring to prevent burning. After 2 minutes turn heat down to low and simmer.

8. Now, put it all together. With a fork, scrape out the spaghetti squash "noodles" into a medium casserole dish. Add the cooked sausage, broccoli, and creamy garlic sauce. Mix everything together well.

9. Place back in the oven to bake for 15 more minutes. Remove and serve.

NUTRITION INFORMATION

Per Serving: **Calories**: 308; **Total Fat**: 22 g; **Saturated Fat**: 9 g; **Monounsaturated Fat**: 0 g; **Polyunsaturated Fat**: 0 g; **Cholesterol**: 51 mg; **Sodium**: 1255 mg; **Potassium**: 204 mg; **Carbohydrate**: 13 g; **Fiber**: 2 g; **Sugar**: 2 g; **Protein**: 20 g

NUTRITION BONUS:

Vitamin C: 36%; **Vitamin A**: 9%; **Iron**: 6%; **Calcium**: 17%;

2. BAKED PARMESAN ZUCCHINI FRIES

Prep time: 5 mins

Cook time: 22 mins

Total time: 27 mins

Your new favorite way to eat zucchini! These Baked Parmesan Zucchini Fries are loaded with flavor and baked to golden perfection! The perfect way to use up your summer bounty!

Recipe type: Dinner

Serves: 4 servings

INGREDIENTS

- 2 medium zucchini
- ½ cup all purpose flour (optional)
- 2 eggs, lightly beaten
- ½ cup Panko bread crumbs
- ¼ cup grated Parmesan cheese
- ¼ tsp salt
- ¼ tsp pepper
- ¼ tsp paprika
- ¼ tsp garlic powder
- ¼ tsp Italian seasoning

INSTRUCTIONS

1. Preheat the oven to 425F.

2. Line a baking sheet with foil and spray with cooking spray.

3. Combine bread crumbs, Parmesan cheese, salt, pepper, paprika, garlic powder and Italian seasoning in a small bowl.

4. Cut off the ends of the zucchini. Cut the zucchini in half and then cut into ½-inch wide stripes or wedges.

5. Coat the zucchini with flour, if desired. This step is optional.

6. Dip the zucchini strips into the beaten egg and shake off excess.

7. Dredge zucchini in the bread crumb mixture and place on the prepared baking sheet.

8. Repeat for all zucchini fries. Spray the top of the zucchini with cooking spray.

9. Bake zucchini fries for 22 to 25 minutes, or until golden brown and crisp. Turn over halfway through.

3. VIETNAMESE CHICKEN SUMMER ROLLS WITH PINEAPPLE BANANA SMOOTHIE

This Vietnamese meal is light and delicious and just takes a little practice. Once you get a hang of making these rolls, you can get creative with any filling under the sun!

Enjoy dipped in classic nuoc nam and enjoy with a tropical smoothie!

Smarts: If you're feeling lazy and don't want to make the rolls, just enjoy this as a noodle bowl with the nuoc nam as a dressing.

INGREDIENTS

- To properly measure aromatics like garlic and onion, check out our guide.
- 4 servings Metric

PINEAPPLE BANANA SMOOTHIE:

- Pineapple - 1/2, chopped
- Bananas - 2
- Frozen strawberries - 2 cups
- Coconut milk - 1 cup ((Or sub plain yogurt))

VIETNAMESE CHICKEN SUMMER ROLLS:

- Rice vermicelli noodles - 4 oz ((Find these thin rice noodles in the ethnic aisle. If you can't find them, substitute with another thin noodle))
- Leftover chicken breasts - 1 lb, sliced
- Cucumbers - 2/3 lb, sliced into matchsticks
- Green lettuce - 4 leaves, torn

- Rice papers - 16 sheets ((You will probably make about 4 to 6 / person. Look for them in the ethnic aisle. They are made from rice or tapioca flour so GF!))

- Leftover grated carrots - 1 cup ((~1 carrot))

- Leftover nuoc nam - 1 cup

4. CILANTRO LIME CHICKEN WINGS

INGREDIENTS

- 2-3 jalapeno peppers, ribs and seeds removed

- 3 garlic cloves, peeled

- 1/2 cup fresh cilantro

- Zest from 2 limes

- 1/4 cup lime juice

- 2 tablespoons soy sauce or coconut aminos

- 1 tablespoon olive oil

- 1 tablespoon raw honey, optional (sugars will cook off from grill but adds a sweetness to the zest)

- 4 pounds chicken wings and/or drumsticks

- 4 limes, for garnish

INSTRUCTIONS

1. Add jalapenos, garlic cloves, fresh cilantro, lime zest, lime juice, soy sauce, olive oil and honey into a blender or food processor to create marinade.

2. Place chicken wings in a bowl or Ziploc bag and mix with marinade. Marinate chicken for 1 hour up to 10 hours (I wouldn't marinate longer than 10 hours because the lime zest has acidity that could break down the chicken which is not tasty)

3. Grill according to your individual grill settings (or bake for 50 minutes in an oven at 400 degrees, flipping halfway through on a baking sheet or broiler pan!)

5. SUMMER KALE ROLLS

Prep Time: 10 minutes

Cook Time: 10-15 minutes

Servings: 2

INGREDIENTS

- 1 tablespoon extra-virgin olive oil
- grated zest and juice of 1/2 lemon
- 1/8 teaspoon ground cumin
- 1/8 teaspoon salt
- 1/8 teaspoon ground black pepper
- 1 pint snap peas
- 2 scallions
- 7-10 mint leaves
- 1/8 cup shelled pistachios, coarsely chopped

INSTRUCTIONS

1. In a large bowl, mix olive oil, lemon juice, cumin, salt, and pepper. Set aside.

2. Cut the snap peas, scallions, and mint leaves into julienne slivers lengthwise and place in the bowl with the dressing.

3. Add the pistachios.

4. Toss to combine.

5. Allow flavors to meld about 10-15 minutes before eating.

NUTRITION INFORMATION

Per Serving: **Calories**: 145;

Total Fat: 11 g; **Saturated Fat**: 2 g; **Monounsaturated Fat**: 7 g; **Polyunsaturated Fat**: 2 g;

Cholesterol: 1 mg; **Sodium**: 45 mg; **Potassium**: 222 mg; **Carbohydrate**: 13 g; **Fiber**: 4 g; **Sugar**: 5 g; **Protein**: 4 g;

Nutrition Bonus: **Vitamin C**: 65%; **Vitamin A**: 20%; **Iron**: 9%; **Calcium**: 5%;

6. SLOW COOKER BUFFALO CHICKEN AND BLUE CHEESE CABBAGE BOWL

Slow Cooker Buffalo Chicken and Blue Cheese Cabbage Bowl is perfect for an easy low-carb and gluten-free summer dinner from the slow Cooker and this tasty bowl meal is also South Beach Diet Phase One. And you can make this tasty bowl meal in the slow cooker or pressure cooker, take your pick!

I think the combination of spicy chicken and cooling coleslaw make this perfect for a Slow Cooker Summer Dinner, and yum, blue cheese!

Makes 4-6 servings

BUFFALO CHICKEN INGREDIENTS:

- 4 boneless, skinless chicken breasts

- 1 cup homemade chicken stock or canned chicken broth

- 1 tsp. Poultry Seasoning

- 1/2 tsp. garlic powder

- 1/2 tsp. onion powder

- 3/4 cup Franks Red Hot Sauce or Frank's Buffalo Wing Sauce

- 2 T olive oil

- 2 T Worcestershire sauce (gluten-free if needed)

- 2 tsp. Green Tabasco sauce or other green hot sauce (optional, but good)

- 1-2 T agave nectar (or other sweetener of your choice)

OTHER INGREDIENTS:

- 6 T thick blue cheese dressing (I like Lighthouse Original Blue Cheese for this.)

- 2-3 T low-fat buttermilk

- 1/2 large head green cabbage, thinly sliced and then chopped

- 1/2 large head red cabbage, thinly sliced and then chopped

- 1/2 cup thickly sliced green onion

- 2 tsp. celery seed

- salt and fresh-ground black pepper to taste

- 1/3 cup crumbled blue cheese for serving + more blue cheese to add to the slaw if desired

INSTRUCTIONS:

1. Trim chicken breasts and cut into half lengthwise. Spray the slow cooker insert with olive oil or non-stick spray and place chicken in the slow cooker. Mix the chicken stock, poultry seasoning, garlic powder, and onion powder and pour over the chicken. Cook on high for about 3 hours or until chicken shreds apart easily with a fork.

2. When chicken is tender, drain in a colander placed in the sink, discarding the stock the chicken was cooked in, or strain the stock and freeze or use in another recipe. Let chicken cool for a few minutes so it's easier to handle, then shred chicken apart with two forks. (You can rinse the chicken before you shred it if you prefer, but I didn't worry about it.) Mix Frank's Hot Sauce, olive oil, Worcestershire sauce, Green Tabasco Sauce, and Agave Nectar or sweetener of your choice.

3. Put the shredded chicken back into the slow cooker and pour the sauce over, stirring gently to combine the chicken and sauce. Cook on high while you follow instructions to prepare Ridiculously Easy Blue Cheese Coleslaw, adding some blue cheese crumbles to the coleslaw mixture if desired.

4. To serve put a generous amount of slaw into a bowl and top with a scoop of the buffalo chicken mixture. Sprinkle crumbled blue cheese over the top and serve. (If this recipe makes more than you'll eat at one time, I recommend refrigerating the cabbage mixture, dressing, and buffalo chicken separately. Then when you want to make a Buffalo Chicken and Blue Cheese Cabbage Bowl heat the chicken, mix some dressing into the slaw, and serve.)

7. DETOX FRIENDLY CAULIFLOWER PIZZA

Prep Time: 15 minutes

Cook Time: 30 minutes

Servings: 6

INGREDIENTS

- For the crust:
- 1/2 head cauliflower
- 2 tbsp almond meal (ground almonds)
- 1 tsp oregano
- 1 egg

For the sauce:

- 1 large tomato
- 1 small squeeze tomato paste (optional)
- 1 head garlic
- 1 handful basil
- 1 drizzle olive oil

For the toppings:

- Handful spinach
- Artichoke hearts

- Zucchini

- Red pepper

- Mushrooms

INSTRUCTIONS

For the crust:

1. Using your food processor or blender, adding your chopped cauliflower to create 'rice' (it should be quite fine).

2. Add to a bowl and microwave 5 minutes, or place on the stove in a pan to cook until soft.

3. Add to a clean kitchen towel and allow to cool, then squeeze out all excess liquid. The more liquid you get out the better it will stay together when cook.

4. Add the rest of your ingredients into a bowl with the cauliflower and mix with your hands until well combined.

5. On a cookie sheet lined with parchment paper, spread your mixture until 2cm thick (roughly).

6. Bake for 20 minutes or until it's lightly browned, at 350F.

For the sauce:

1. Blend all ingredients until smooth.

2. Add to your pan on the stove and cook until heated through.

3. After your pizza crust has been in the oven and is cooked, take out and add the sauce.

To assemble:

1. Chop your hearts, zucchini, mushrooms and red pepper.

2. Add to a pan with a dash of water and cook for 2 minutes until slightly tender.

3. This will help the cooking process on the pizza.

4. Add all ingredients + spinach on top of your pizza sauce then place back in the oven another 5 minutes.

5. Allow to cool before eating.

NUTRITION INFORMATION

Per Serving:

Calories: 76; **Total Fat**: 3 g; **Saturated Fat**: 1 g; **Monounsaturated Fat**: 1 g; **Polyunsaturated Fat**: 0 g; **Cholesterol**: 31 mg; **Sodium**: 100 mg; **Potassium**: 424 mg;

Carbohydrate: 9 g; **Fiber**: 3 g; **Sugar**: 4 g; **Protein**: 5 g

Nutrition Bonus:

Vitamin C: 97%; **Vitamin A**: 26%; **Iron**: 7%; **Calcium**: 5%;

8. SRIRACHA HONEY SPARERIBS

Servings: 6

Prep Time: 10minutes

Cook Time: 21/4hours

Passive Time: 3hours

INGREDIENTS

- 5-6 lbs. pork spareribs or 3-4 lbs. country style ribs

- salt and pepper

- 4 oranges

- 2 tbsp sriracha sauce (or to taste) preferably one without additives and preservatives; see note.

- 2 tbsp honey

- 2 tbsp rice wine vinegar

- 2 tbsp Worcestershire sauce

- 2 cloves garlic or shallot minced

Instructions

1. Preheat oven to 350 degrees F. Prepare the ribs by removing the membrane on the back of the ribs. Using a small, sharp knife, start on one corner and cut under the membrane until you have enough to grasp with a paper towel. Pull the membrane steadily away and towards the opposite end of the ribs. You can often remove the whole thing in two

or three strips. Be sure to do this so the glaze will be absorbed into all the meat.

2. Separate the ribs into 2-rib sections and generously salt and pepper. Arrange the ribs on an aluminum foil covered baking sheet in a single layer, using two sheets if necessary.

3. Bake for 45 minutes. Meanwhile prepare glaze.

4. Remove the orange peel in long strips. You should have some pith on each strip as this gives the glaze its punch. Thinly slice the peels into long julienne slices and place in saucepan. Juice the oranges and add juice and pulp to saucepan.

5. Add all the remaining ingredients and bring to a simmer over medium heat. Allow to reduce until the mixture bubbles and get syrupy, about 5-7 minutes. Taste for balance adding additional sriracha, honey, vinegar and/ or Worcestershire so the glaze is to your liking.

6. When the 45 minutes is up, turn off the oven. Spoon the glaze over the ribs, making sure to cover both sides. Return the ribs to oven. Allow to rest without additional heat for 3 hours. (If you want to cook the ribs in two stages, do not return the ribs to the turned-off oven, but allow them to reach room temperature. Refrigerate until you want to resume cooking - great if you want to serve the ribs on a weeknight and don't have time during the day to do the initial prep.)

7. Heat the oven to 325 degrees F. You do not need to preheat. Roast the ribs for 1 1/2 hours (rotating the baking sheets and switching racks after 45 minutes). Serve and enjoy!

9. LEMON HERB SALMON PATTIES

INGREDIENTS:

- 1lb raw salmon, skin removed
- 1 egg + 1 egg white, lightly beaten
- 1 cup almond flour (I used Bob's Red Mill)
- 1/4 cup chopped fresh parsley
- 1/4 cup chopped fresh basil
- 1/4 red or yellow onion, finely diced (as tiny as possible!)
- 2 cloves of garlic, minced
- 1/4 tsp dried marjoram
- 1/4 tsp onion powder
- juice of 1 lemon (If you only use 1/2, the lemon flavor doesn't shine through)
- salt and pepper

INSTRUCTIONS:

1. In the bowl of a food processor, add the raw salmon and pulse until it's evenly ground and starting to be sticky.

2. Combine all the remaining ingredients in a bowl and add the salmon. Mix to combine. Lightly score the mixture into 4 sections. Form the 4 pieces into burger patties.

3. Add a little bit of olive oil to the bottom of a large skillet over medium-high heat. Once the oil is hot, add the salmon patties and cook for about 4 minutes per side. Remove when they're cooked through and no longer pink. Enjoy!

Servings: 4.

Approximate Nutritional Information per Serving:

Calories: 364; **Carbs**: 3g; **Fat**: 23g; **Protein**: 32g; **Fiber**: 3g; **Points+**: 9 Recipe adapted from here.

For the homemade ranch-style sauce:

- 1 egg
- 1 cup extra light (must be extra light!) olive oil
- 1 tablespoon lemon juice
- 1/2 tbsp apple cider vinegar
- 1/4 tsp salt
- 1/2 tsp dried dill
- 1 tsp onion powder
- 1/2 tsp dried parsley
- 1/4 tsp garlic powder
- 1/2 tsp lime juice (optional)
- 1 jalapeno, seeded and minced (optional)
- Salt and pepper, to taste.
- Immersion blender

DIRECTIONS:

1. Important: You will need an immersion blender to do this. Place the egg, olive oil, lemon juice, vinegar, and salt into a mason jar or container with tall sides. Put the immersion blender in the container so it's resting at the very bottom, then turn it on. Let it blend like this for several seconds, then slowly and gently move it up so it blends all of the mixture. This should take less than a minute.

2. Once it's blended through, add the remaining ingredients and stir together. Cover and refrigerate for up to 2 weeks! If you want to make it into a thinner dressing, add a tiny bit of water at a time and stir until you get the consistency you want.

10. QUICK CAULIFLOWER COCONUT STEW

Prep Time: 10 minutes

Cook Time: 35 minutes

Servings: 4

Ingredients

- 2 tablespoons coconut oil
- 1 teaspoon cumin seeds
- 1 medium onion, finely chopped
- 3 ripe tomatoes, finely chopped
- 1 medium head cauliflower, stemmed and cut into bite-size florets
- 1 jalapeno, stemmed, seeded, chopped
- 1 can full-fat, unsweetened coconut milk
- 1 cup chopped kale
- 2 tablespoons chopped cilantro
- 1 tablespoon cumin powder
- 1 tablespoon coriander powder
- 2 teaspoons ginger paste
- 1 teaspoon turmeric powder
- 1 teaspoon sea salt

INSTRUCTIONS

1. In a medium stock pot, heat the coconut oil for 30 seconds on medium heat.

2. Add the cumin seeds and stir until they start to sputter. Then add the onions and cook for another minute, and then, add the tomatoes, stir and cook for a few more minutes until the tomatoes soften.

3. Add the rest of the ingredients and stir together. Cover the pan and simmer for about 15 minutes, stirring every 5 minutes to keep from burning.

4. Ladle the soup into 4 serving bowls and enjoy! Leftover stew can be stored in air-tight container and saved for lunch the next day.

NUTRITION INFORMATION

Per Serving:

Calories: 140; **Total Fat**: 10 g; **Saturated Fat**: 8 g; **Monounsaturated Fat**: 1 g; **Polyunsaturated Fat**: 1 g; **Cholesterol**: 0 mg; **Sodium**: 525 mg; **Potassium**: 576 mg;

Carbohydrate: 14 g; **Fiber**: 4 g; **Sugar**: 6 g; **Protein**: 4 g

Nutrition Bonus:

Vitamin C: 143%; **Vitamin A**: 18%; **Iron**: 8%; **Calcium**: 27%;

CONCLUSION

Carb cycling may be a useful tool for those trying to optimize their diet, physical performance and health.

The individual mechanisms behind carb cycling are supported by research. However, no direct research has investigated a long-term carb cycling diet.

Rather than chronic low or high-carb diets, a balance between the two may be beneficial from both a physiological and psychological perspective.

If using carb cycling for fat loss, ensure that your protein intake is adequate and you maintain a calorie deficit.

Always experiment with the protocol and amounts of carbohydrates to find the best fit for you.

Made in the USA
San Bernardino, CA
14 February 2018